Maximizing Benefits with Vitamin D, Vitamin C, and Iodine

A Comprehensive Guide to a Healthier You

Brenda F. Dozier

Table of content

Introduction

Iodine, vitamin D, and vitamin C are three of the few substances that stand out as unquestionable protagonists in the mosaic of human health, where every nutrient plays an important part with equal importance. In addition to the fact that their names are well-known, these nutritional powerhouses are responsible for weaving elaborate stories inside the physiology of our bodies. They conduct a symphony of well-being that goes far beyond the limitations of a vitamin pill.

Imagine that vitamin D is the sunbeam conductor, responsible for conducting a melodious dance with our skin cells and changing the mundane into the exceptional. In this symphony, each ray transforms into a cascade of biological reactions, bolstering bones, energizing the immune system, and throwing away the shadows of deficiency that linger on the horizon of health.

Then there is the vivacious soloist that is vitamin C, which is a powerful antioxidant that comes into the spotlight and brandishes its shield against the unrelenting assault of oxidative stress. By strengthening immune defenses, promoting collagen synthesis for increased skin suppleness, and leaving an indelible mark on the canvas of cellular resilience, it fights a gallant war with each molecule that it produces.

Moreover, in order to avoid being overshadowed, iodine appears as the unsung hero, as it is responsible for maintaining the delicate equilibrium of thyroid function. It is common to underestimate the importance of this micronutrient, which serves as the silent architect of metabolic harmony. It ensures a flawless interaction between the production of energy, the regulation of temperature, and the maintenance of hormonal equilibrium.

On the other hand, the strengths of these components are not limited to their unique capabilities. The alchemy lies in their combined resonance, as they participate in a harmonious ballet within our bodies. Creating a comprehensive tapestry of well-being is the result of the dynamic three of vitamin D, vitamin C, and iodine working together in a ballet of health. They complement and enhance each other's effects to provide a more complete picture of health.

As we travel the hallways of this thorough guide, expect to find the mysteries contained in the biochemical poetry of these vitamins and minerals. Through research and disclosure, we will unravel the tales of resilience, immunological fortification, and metabolic balance that these nutrients inscribe upon the pages of our biological narrative. It's time to begin on a trip below the surface, into the profound symphony of Vitamin D, Vitamin C, and Iodine—a symphony that resonates with the very essence of a healthier, more vibrant self.

Unveiling the Importance of Vitamins in Health

In the wonderful chronicle of human health, vitamins appear as the unsung architects, delicately crafting the cornerstone of our well-being. Consider these critical nutrients as the attentive custodians of vitality, each playing a particular role in the constant drama of our physiological homeostasis.

Vitamins, sometimes considered ordinary supplements, are the maestros orchestrating the symphony of life within our bodies. Their significance stretches far beyond the bounds of regular eating routines; they are the clandestine builders constructing the fundamental infrastructure of our health. In this magnificent theater, each vitamin adopts a unique character, adding to a drama that transcends the routine and journeys into the world of amazing resistance.

Consider Vitamin A as the virtuoso of vision, painting the canvas of our retinas with hues of clarity. A lack, equivalent to lowering the lights, interrupts the visual masterpiece, underscoring the important function played by this vitamin in preserving eye health.

Vitamin E, the custodian of cellular sanctuaries, acts as a sturdy defender against the onslaught of oxidative stress. It is the unsung hero, softly patrolling our cellular landscapes and defending delicate membranes from the ravages of free radicals.

The B-vitamin ensemble, with its various casts including B1, B2, B3, and beyond, takes center stage in metabolic ballet. This troupe controls the energy orchestra, guaranteeing the flawless transformation of nutrients into the vital life force that propels us ahead.

In this unfolding of the vitamin narrative, we observe the immense impact of these microcosmic beings on our macroscopic existence. They are the architects of resilience, the sentinels guarding against the degradation of health, and the catalysts propelling us towards the apex of well-being. As we walk the corridors of this exploration, the relevance of vitamins in health reveals itself not as a minor subplot but as the very essence of a thriving, vibrant existence—a life where each vitamin plays a role, not merely in supporting us but in elevating us to our most robust, radiant selves.

The Dynamic Trio: Vitamin D, Vitamin C, and Iodine

Regard the human body as a magnificent symphony, with each note harmonizing with the next to produce a masterpiece of vitality. Amidst this orchestration, a trio of vital actors emerges: vitamin D, vitamin C, and iodine. These three virtuosos, diverse in their responsibilities, converge to form a vibrant tune that resonates across the hallways of holistic health.

Vitamin D, the dazzling conductor, takes center stage, orchestrating a solar ballet with the skin as its stage. Sunlight, the maestro's baton, instigates a dance that exceeds mere warmth, instilling bones with power and reinforcing the immune system with a crescendo of resilience. In this cosmic ballet, Vitamin D is not only a nutrient; it is the sunbeam symphony that transforms the ordinary into the spectacular.

Enter Vitamin C, the virtuoso soloist wielding the baton against the continuous onslaught of oxidative stress. This antioxidant champion plays a critical role in cellular defense and is a sturdy defender against the wear and tear of time. Its presence is not simply a shield; it's an anthem of immunity, a symphony that resonates through tissues and organs, constructing a protective layer against the tiny symphonies of aging.

Iodine, the unsung hero, enters the limelight with quiet authority, guaranteeing the delicate balance of thyroid function. This micronutrient, frequently ignored, builds a rich narrative of metabolic stability, directing the delicate interplay between energy generation, temperature regulation, and hormonal balance. Iodine is not just a footnote in the health text; it is the quiet architect of the body's metabolic masterwork.

Together, this dynamic trio builds a symphony of health, with each nutrient playing an essential note in the composition of vitality. Their collaboration is not a happenstance but an intentional arrangement in the musical score of wellbeing. Vitamin D, Vitamin C, and Iodine—the architects of resilience, the conductors of immunity, and the silent orchestrators of metabolic harmony—are not just ingredients; they are the song, the rhythm, and the harmony of a flourishing life.

Chapter 1

The Sunshine Vitamin - Vitamin D

Imagine Vitamin D as the enigmatic maestro in the symphony of human health—a maestro who orchestrates a bright ballet upon the canvas of our skin. This sunshine vitamin, considerably more than basic food, is a brilliant energy that transforms the commonplace act of basking in sunlight into an astonishing composition of well-being. In this cosmic ballet, sunshine becomes the conductor's baton, while Vitamin D, the lead actor, casts a transformational spell upon the body.

Picture the skin as a responsive stage, where every sunbeam is a note, and Vitamin D is the melody that fortifies bones and invigorates the immune system. It is not only a nutrient; it is the manifestation of a sunny symphony that echoes through the very sinews of our existence. Beyond its role in calcium absorption, Vitamin D becomes the radiant conductor of resilience, establishing a crescendo of power within the skeletal framework and harmonizing the immunological response to a melody of invincibility.

This luminous force reaches beyond the tangible, delving into the delicate world of mood management. Vitamin D, like a guardian angel, regulates the synthesis of serotonin, the neurotransmitter associated with mood and well-being. It is not only a vitamin; it is the sunny troubadour serenading the mind with notes of positivity and mental stability.

Yet, the drama of vitamin D only occurs under the sun's limelight. It is an ongoing narrative within our bodies, a tale of balance and synthesis. In the labyrinthine pathways of metabolism, vitamin D assumes the role of a versatile protagonist, affecting gene expression and contributing to a complex network of physiological interactions.

As the sun ascends in the sky, Vitamin D unfurls its luminous wings, commencing on a transforming trip through our bodies. It's the conductor of a metabolic opera, where each note vibrates with the rhythm of life. The skin, more than a plain surface, becomes a sunlit stage, and Vitamin D takes center stage in a bright performance that surpasses the limitations of a nutrient and journeys into the realm of physiological poetry.

The crossing of Vitamin D extends into the bones, where it choreographs a dance of power and resilience. This sunlight virtuoso boosts calcium absorption, reinforcing the skeletal structure and producing a crescendo of toughness. It's the architect of bone density, ensuring that the body's foundation stands solid against the winds of fragility.

In the symphony of immunity, Vitamin D conducts a melody of defense. It orchestrates a harmonic interplay between distinct immune cells, fine-tuning their reactions to external threats. This vitamin, bathed in the sunlight's brilliance, becomes the sentinel of resistance, warding off the shadows of illnesses and reinforcing the body's natural defense mechanisms.

Yet, the bright narrative doesn't conclude there. Vitamin D, the brilliant maestro, expands its effect to the complicated domain of genetics. It controls gene expression, shaping the physiological reactions that ripple across the body's genetic fabric. This is not a static nutrient; it's a dynamic force, telling a nuanced tale of adaptability and equilibrium.

As we go deeper into the sunny domain of Vitamin D, it becomes obvious that this substance is not bound to a specific job. It is the radiant storyteller, narrating a history of bone health, immunological fortification, and genetic orchestration. It's the sunlight that transforms the skin into a resonant canvas, painting an image of energy that exceeds the ordinary knowledge of a vitamin. Vitamin D is not only a nutrient; it is the dazzling power that orchestrates the magnificent symphony of our physiological well-being.

Understanding Vitamin D and Its Sources

Visualize a small sun, not in the sky, but pulsing through your veins. That's vitamin D, a fun nutrient as colorful as its source. Unlike others, Vitamin D bypasses the grocery store, preferring a DIY approach. When your skin waltzes with sunshine, it triggers a hidden factory, churning forth this amazing elixir. It's a monument to the body's resourcefulness, creating its own wellness potion from a divine embrace.

But vitamin D's magic isn't just about sunbathing. It's a bone builder extraordinaire, setting down calcium bricks like a master architect. This translates to strong bones, standing tall against osteoporosis, the silent thief of mobility. Vitamin D is also the cheerleader of immunity, mobilizing white blood cell troops against invaders. It sharpens their weapons, enhances their spirit, and transforms them into an invincible force defending their health.

But wait, there's more! Vitamin D is like a mood maestro, painting sunshine on your emotions. It chases away the shadows of despair and anxiety, letting your inner sun shine brightly. It's a natural pick-me-up, a ray of light that removes the fog and let's joy blossom.

Now, while sunshine is Vitamin D's playground, it's not the only game in town. Fatty fish like salmon and tuna offer their own golden treasure, and even mushrooms caressed by sunlight have their part. And for individuals living under overcast skies, fortified foods like milk and cereals come in as vitamin D buddies.

But sometimes, even with good intentions, our vitamin D levels can decrease. Fatigue, achy bones, and a bad mood can be whispers of a concealed insufficiency. A simple blood test can disclose the truth, and your doctor can become your Vitamin D navigator, guiding you towards sunshine, dietary modifications, or even a supplement—ensuring your superhero within receives the fuel it needs.

So, the next time you feel the sun's warm kiss, remember the secret sunshine within you. Vitamin D, a gift from the sky, offers a promise of vigor, resilience, and well-being. Let its light guide you, and together, you'll create a fortress of health, one sunbeam at a time.

Remember, while sunshine is a great ally, moderation is crucial. Seek shade during peak hours, and wear sunscreen to protect your skin. And if you have concerns, always visit your doctor.

Embrace the sunshine, both within and without, and let Vitamin D brighten your road to a vibrant life!

The Role of Sunlight in Vitamin D Synthesis

Bathed in the ethereal glow of sunlight, the skin becomes more than a protective barrier—it turns into a key component in a sunny ballet of biological alchemy. The significance of sunshine in vitamin D production is nothing short of spectacular, brilliant cooperation that unfolds each time sunlight caresses the skin's surface.

At the core of this celestial choreography lies 7-dehydrocholesterol, a molecule dwelling in the skin's depths. When exposed to the sun's ultraviolet B (UVB) rays, this inconspicuous molecule undergoes a metamorphosis, beginning a molecular dance that sets the stage for vitamin D synthesis. It's a cosmic waltz where sunlight becomes the spark for change, beginning a cascade of reactions that eventually create vitamin D3.

As this forerunner evolves, it becomes the protagonist in a sunny drama. The skin, serving as a natural solar sensor, catches the radiance supplied by sunlight and directs it into a biological masterpiece. This is not passive absorption; it's an active collaboration between the skin and the sun, a partnership that exceeds the mundane knowledge of human anatomy.

The process doesn't finish with the production of vitamin D3. Nature, in its exquisite simplicity, has fashioned a finale where body heat completes the synthesis. The skin, warmed by the body's inner glow, pushes the final change, transforming pre-vitamin D3 into the active form of vitamin D. It's a symphony of sunlight and warmth, where every note adds to the synthesis of a nutrient important for skeletal strength, immune resistance, and overall well-being.

In the brilliant mix of sunlight and skin, we see not merely a biochemical process but a choreographed dance of life. It's a tale where sunshine becomes the conductor, the skin the responsive stage, and Vitamin D the dazzling protagonist. This is not only a scientific term; it's a harmonious union between the cosmic and the corporeal—a dance of light that surpasses the limitations of our ordinary awareness.

Health Impacts of Vitamin D Deficiency

Picture the body as a perfectly tuned instrument, where each nutrient plays a keynote in the symphony of health. When the melody of Vitamin D is absent or subdued owing to lack, the repercussions ricochet across the physiological score, hitting not only the bones but weaving a tale of future health concerns.

Foremost among these consequences is that the skeletal symphony is disturbed. Vitamin D, the conductor of calcium absorption, orchestrates the fortification of bones and teeth. In its absence, the harmony falters, leading to a crescendo of consequences—brittle bones, a heightened risk of fractures, and a disorder known as rickets in infants and osteocalcin in adults. This is more than a weakening of the structural foundation; it's a devastating sonnet of fragility inscribed into the very architecture of the body.

Yet, the ramifications extend beyond the skeleton stage. Vitamin D insufficiency puts a shadow over the immune system, diminishing its robustness. The immunological symphony, carefully tuned by radiant nutrition, loses its vigor, rendering the body susceptible to illnesses and impairing its ability to mount a defense. It's a vulnerability that echoes through the hallways of health, leaving the body prone to a spectrum of illnesses.

In the psychological sphere, vitamin D insufficiency adds a gloomy undertone. The radiant nutrient is not merely a conductor of physical health; it also influences emotions and mental well-being. Its absence has been related to an increased risk of mood disorders, including depression. It's a discord in mental harmony where the absence of Vitamin D becomes a silent contributor to the symphony of psychological issues.

The cardiovascular system, too, feels the impact. Vitamin D insufficiency has been associated with a higher risk of heart-related disorders, adding a dismal note to the cardiovascular makeup. It's a reminder that the brilliance of this vitamin extends beyond the evidence, reaching into the intricate networks of the body's critical systems.

From the perspective of health, vitamin D deficiency is not only an absence of a vitamin; it's a disruption in the orchestration of well-being. It's a story where bones lose their tenacity, the immune system falters, moods lose their brilliance, and the cardiovascular rhythm slips. The health repercussions of Vitamin D deficiency constitute a heartbreaking melody of fragility, reminding us that in the absence of this dazzling mineral, the symphony of health may play a mournful tune

Chapter 2

The Immunity Booster - Vitamin C

Vitamin C is the undeniable immunity booster, a caped crusader in the continuous war against invading viruses, and it appears as the most powerful nutritional superhero in the broad spectrum of potential nutritional superheroes. This essential nutrient is not merely a defender; rather, it is the vigilant guardian that strengthens the immune defenses of the body, carrying out a symphony of resilience that reverberates into the very core of our well-being.

Imagine that vitamin C is the conductor of a musical defense against the effects of oxidative stress. Free radicals are rogue agents that strive to destroy cellular peace. This antioxidant powerhouse acts as a shield, neutralizing free radicals and preventing them from doing so. It is a fierce protector that fights against the wear and tear that is imposed upon the body by the unrelenting forces of time and the stressors that come from the outside world.

Vitamin C, in addition to its function as an antioxidant, also plays the role of a strategic commander within the immune system. It does this by enhancing the effectiveness of immune cells, from the steadfast phagocytes to the flexible lymphocytes, making certain that they function at the highest possible level of their capacities. Vitamin C is responsible for orchestrating a harmonic response during times of microbial invasion, which aids in strengthening the body's ability to defend itself against infections and disorders.

However, this is not the end of the story about immunity-boosting. The synthesis and function of white blood cells, which are the first line of defense in the immunological defense army, are both improved by vitamin C, which is brilliant in many different ways. It's a vitamin that not only provides the arsenal but also sharpens the precision of the immune system's weaponry, producing a robust line of defense against intruders.

Beyond its immunological capabilities, Vitamin C contributes to the manufacture of collagen, the structural protein that weaves the fabric of skin, blood vessels, and connective tissues. It becomes a regenerative force, not merely bolstering the immune defenses but also nourishing the body's architectural integrity.

In the vast canvas of health, Vitamin C is not just a nutrient; it is the virtuoso immune booster, orchestrating a symphony of defense that defies the mundane idea of a vitamin. It's the guardian of well-being, the defender against the wear and tear of time, and the composer of a resilient symphony that resonates through the immunological corridors, ensuring the body's ability to stand strong against the obstacles that come its way.

Exploring the Antioxidant Power of Vitamin C

In the cosmic ballet of human health, Vitamin C appears not simply as a source of nutrition but as a brilliant force—a beacon of antioxidant potency that orchestrates a symphony of cellular defense. Picture this crucial nutrient as a sentry, keeping guard against the unrelenting onslaught of free radicals, those wayward agents that threaten to destroy the delicate harmony within our cells.

Vitamin C, in its antioxidant brilliance, becomes the protector against oxidative stress, a tremendous force unleashed by events ranging from pollution to the natural process of aging. It's analogous to a shield, intercepting and neutralizing the free radicals that strive to wreak havoc on our cellular landscape. This vitamin becomes a protector of cellular holiness, ensuring that the molecular music within our bodies plays on undisturbed.

Beyond its role as a mere protector, Vitamin C is the alchemist that regenerates and rejuvenates. It contributes electrons to neutralize free radicals, not simply halting the damage but also commencing a process of cellular rejuvenation. In this waltz of electrons, Vitamin C becomes the catalyst for a cascade of defensive processes, reinforcing the cellular architecture and imbuing it with resilience.

Consider this vitamin as a repair maestro, fixing the wear and tear imposed upon the body by the passage of time and environmental stressors. It's the backstage craftsman, stitching together the fabric of connective tissues and stimulating the manufacture of collagen, the protein that provides flexibility to the skin. In this position, vitamin C becomes not merely an antioxidant but a regenerative factor, contributing to the vibrancy and suppleness of our tissues.

The antioxidant power of Vitamin C is beyond its limits of mere protection; it is a dynamic force that engages in a biochemical ballet, maintaining the integrity and vitality of our cells. It's not simply a nutrient; it's a radiant protector, a reparative alchemist, and a guardian of cellular well-being. In the symphony of antioxidants, Vitamin C emerges as the virtuoso, balancing cellular defenses and bolstering the body against the subtle strains of time and environmental obstacles.

Sources and Recommended Daily Intake

In the palette of nutritional abundance, Vitamin C makes its way into our daily lives through an array of sources, each adding to the colorful symphony of health. From the orchards to the ocean's abundance, these sources offer a plethora of alternatives, allowing us to fill our diets with this critical component in a variety of tasty ways.

Citrus fruits, those zesty champions of Vitamin C, rise tall in the orchard's wealth. Oranges, lemons, grapefruits—they're not just zesty joys but also potent transporters of this crucial vitamin. A modest squeeze of lemon into a morning glass of water becomes a delicious elixir of Vitamin C, infusing the day with a rush of tangy power.

Venturing into the vegetable kingdom, bell peppers appear as colorful Vitamin C champions, with hues that range from green to red. These colorful pods pack a punch, delivering not just a delicious crunch to salads but also a substantial dose of immune-boosting benefits.

Strawberries, those ruby-red jewels of deliciousness, become more than just a tantalizing treat for the taste receptors. They are nature's dessert, rich in Vitamin C and antioxidants, merging delight with nourishment in one bite.

For those who love the briny delights of the ocean, seafood provides an alternate outlet. Oysters, a delicacy from the sea, become not simply a culinary joy but also a source of Vitamin C, weaving marine goodness into our nutritional repertory.

As we stroll the aisles of the grocery store, we find fortified foods and new products that bridge the gap between traditional sources and contemporary convenience. From cereals to fruit juices, these fortified treats offer a practical approach to enhancing our diets with Vitamin C, making them more accessible to those with various culinary preferences.

Recommended daily consumption becomes the compass in our nutritional voyage, directing us toward an ideal balance. The daily dose, a compass tuned to individual needs, hangs around 90 mg for men and 75 mg for women. However, this is not a hard prescription; it's a guideline that allows personalization based on age, lifestyle, and overall health.

In the arena of vitamin C, sources become not simply vitamin stores but lively contributors to the culinary canvas.

It's a journey where we can derive this necessary nutrient from a diversity of appetizing options, converting the pursuit of health into a flavorful adventure.

Immune System Support and Beyond

Beyond being the virtuoso of immune system support, Vitamin C unfurls its diverse skill into a plethora of physiological areas, becoming more than just a guardian; it turns into a proactive force in the symphony of general well-being. Visualize it as a multi-faceted jewel, with each facet expressing a different component of health.

In the cosmic dance of antioxidants, Vitamin C steps into the forefront, becoming the defender against oxidative stress. Beyond its immune-boosting activity, it becomes a custodian of cellular integrity, shielding our biological architecture from the insidious onslaught of free radicals. It's a vitamin that not only bolsters our immune systems but also fortifies the very fabric of our cellular resistance.

Consider the skin, the body's outermost tapestry, where Vitamin C becomes the maestro of collagen synthesis. It is the invisible architect weaving the structural proteins that offer elasticity and suppleness. In this position, Vitamin C becomes more than an immunological ally; it transforms into a guardian of skin health, contributing to the brightness and resilience that radiate from within.

The cardiovascular symphony finds a harmonious note in the action of Vitamin C. As an antioxidant, it aids in the maintenance of arterial health, decreasing oxidative stress that could compromise cardiovascular well-being. It is not only an immune supporter; it becomes a cardiovascular ally, navigating the complicated pathways of heart health.

The restorative role extends to Vitamin C's partnership with iron absorption. By boosting the absorption of non-heme iron from plant-based sources, it becomes a facilitator of iron metabolism, maintaining the body's supply of this crucial element. In this alliance, Vitamin C becomes more than an immunological sentinel; it transforms into a major component in the rich tapestry of nutritional synergy.

In the orchestra of health, Vitamin C, with its far-reaching influence, becomes a conductor, orchestrating not just immunological resilience but a symphony of total well-being. It is a multifaceted diamond, blazing bright in the different facets of health—from cellular defense to skin vitality and nutritional equilibrium. In comprehending Vitamin C, we unravel not just a nutrient but a dynamic force that adds to the thriving song of a healthy and lively life.

Chapter 3

Iodine - Essential for Thyroid Health

Nestled deep in the neck, the thyroid gland acts like a silent director, orchestrating the symphony of your metabolism. It fuels your energy, regulates your heart, and even influences your emotions, but it needs a tiny spark to ignite this vibrant performance: iodine.

Think of iodine as the conductor's baton, hammering out the rhythm of your internal orchestra. It's crucial for the creation of thyroid hormones, the chemical messengers that direct the tempo of your body. Without adequate iodine, the orchestra stumbles, notes falter, and the symphony of your health falls out of tune.

This isn't simply about avoiding slow mornings or feeling chilly all the time. Iodine shortage can lead to a cascade of changes, from fatigue and weight gain to brain fog and even goiter, a visible enlargement of the thyroid gland. It's like a butterfly effect, a single missing element generating a cascade of unbalance across your well-being.

But worry not, fellow maestro! Iodine is easily available, waiting to be woven into the fabric of your daily tune. Seaweed whispers its briny secrets, adding a touch of iodine to your sushi or miso soup. Dairy products, like milk and cheese, sing their creamy song, each bite a hushed harmony of critical nutrients. And let's not forget the simple iodized salt, the unsung hero of balanced thyroid function, silently lending its charm to every dish.

So, the next time you grab a bowl of creamy yogurt or sprinkle salt on your roasted vegetables, remember, you're not just adding flavor; you're tuning the delicate melody of your health. You're providing the conductor, your thyroid, the tools it needs to lead, ensuring your internal orchestra plays a lively symphony of well-being.

Remember, iodine is more than simply a mineral; it's a conductor's baton, a butterfly's wing, and a little spark that lights the glorious orchestra of your health. So, keep the baton tapping, keep the symphony playing, and nourish your thyroid with the magic of iodine for a life that hums with lively harmony!

The Crucial Role of Iodine in Thyroid Function

Imagine your body as a sleek, high-powered engine, purring with life. But what if this engine stuttered and coughed, its once-smooth hum replaced by a wobbly chug? It can be missing a critical sparkplug—iodine, the hidden hero of thyroid health.

Tucked up in your neck, the thyroid gland operates like the engine's control center, regulating your metabolism, energy levels, and even body temperature. But it needs fuel to run, and that fuel is iodine. This little mineral, found in oceans and sprinkled in common foods, is the missing piece that ignites the fire within.

Without enough iodine, the thyroid sputters. It struggles to manufacture critical hormones, resulting in a cascade of complications. Fatigue drags you down, your energy level lowers like a collapsing balloon, and your mood could turn as bleak as a rainy day. Brain fog comes in, and even your body temperature struggles to stay stable, leaving you feeling cold even in a warm setting.

But don't fret! This is not a permanent engine breakdown. You can stoke the fire and get your thyroid buzzing again.

Iodine, the missing sparkplug, is readily available in a treasure trove of delectable possibilities. From the briny whisper of seaweed in your sushi to the creamy chorus of milk and cheese, each bite provides a dash of this vital mineral. And let's not forget the simple iodized salt, the silent custodian of thyroid health, silently sprinkling its magic on every meal.

So, the next time you go for a cup of yogurt or season your salad, remember, that you're not simply adding flavor; you're giving your engine the spark it needs to roar. You're guaranteeing your thyroid control center operates efficiently, keeping your body's temperature gauge stable, and your energy levels soaring.

Iodine might be little, but it's the spark that fires the engine of your well-being. Keep the gasoline flowing, listen to the purr of your restored engine, and enjoy the smooth, vibrant ride of optimal health!

Remember, a balanced diet rich in iodine is your best bet for a happy thyroid. If you have any concerns, see your healthcare provider for specialized guidance. Now, go forth and fuel your engine for a life that's full of vitality and zest!

Dietary Sources and Iodine Deficiency

Enter the culinary scene, where the quest for iodine becomes a vivid gastronomic adventure. Amid the abundance of the sea, iodine-rich treasures emerge—seaweeds, that aquatic delicacy, serve as guardians of this crucial element. From nori to kelp, these marine marvels become not just delectable partners to sushi but also a nutritional bridge to appropriate iodine levels.

In the meadows and gardens, the iodine narrative takes on a terrestrial twist. Iodine, absorbed by plants from the soil, manifests in the form of leafy greens and vegetables. Spinach, kale, and potatoes become not just culinary staples but also contributors to our iodine intake. It's a symphony where the soil's iodine whispers find expression in the brilliant hues of our vegetable patches.

Venturing into the animal kingdom, the marine choir continues their singing. Fish, especially those that live in iodine-rich waters, embody the essence of this crucial nutrient. Cod, tuna, and shrimp become not simply exquisite alternatives for the palette but also conduits for preserving iodine equilibrium in the body.

However, the dietary landscape isn't without its obstacles. In some places, where the soil lacks iodine, crops may reflect this paucity, leading to a shortfall in the nutritional supply. The sylvan wealth may not always be sufficient, and in such circumstances, fortification and augmentation become significant notes in the nutritional score.

Iodine insufficiency, when the symphony falters, can cast a shadow over thyroid health. The thyroid, in its hunt for iodine, may expand, giving rise to a condition known as goiter. This visual signal becomes a heartbreaking reminder of the delicate dance between diet and thyroid well-being.

Yet, the perspective is not one of despair but of awareness. It is a culinary head where varied sources can supplement our meals with iodine, ensuring the thyroid's peaceful dance. It's a nutritional story where the sea, the soil, and the plate combine in a gastronomic celebration that goes beyond flavor, nourishing the body and preserving the thyroid's rhythmic energy.

Maintaining Optimal Thyroid Health

Imagine the thyroid as a guardian, a sentinel standing at the crossroads of metabolic vitality, and optimal thyroid health as the symphony it conducts—a harmonious interplay between lifestyle choices and nutrients.

In the culinary realm, the melody begins with diversity. Embrace the riches of the sea, inviting iodine-rich friends like seaweed into your diet. Allow leafy greens and vegetables to color your dish, drawing from the terrestrial iodine wealth cultivated by the soil. Enlist the marine choir, with fish as its vocalists, to imitate the iodine symphony. It's not just about food; it's about creating a nutritious serenade that connects with thyroid well-being.

In this melodious voyage, awareness becomes the conductor's wand. Acknowledge the iodine balance, noting that both lack and excess can affect the thyroid's rhythm. Strike a harmonious chord by embracing a diet that reflects the different note of iodine-rich foods.

The lifestyle overture has a key impact. Bask in the sunlight, allowing the skin's photoreceptors to dance with Vitamin D synthesis—a nutrient that compliments the thyroid's vitality.

Engage in frequent exercise, a rhythmic cadence that reverberates through metabolic pathways, supporting the thyroid's energetic performance.

Amid this symphony, stress becomes a discordant note to be cognizant of. Integrate stress management practices—a meditation minuet or a yoga sonata—to soothe the adrenal crescendo, preventing its echoes from upsetting the thyroid's beautiful song.

As the concluding crescendo in this thyroid opus, consider frequent check-ups. Allow the conductor, your healthcare professional, to examine the thyroid's performance and ensure that the symphony unfolds without conflict.

In the symphony of sustaining optimal thyroid health, the script is not rigorous, and each individual's dietary and lifestyle composition adds a distinctive note. It's a tailored orchestration where awareness and intention become the virtuoso, guiding the thyroid's beautiful melody—a serenade to the rhythm of metabolic well-being.

Chapter 4

The Synergy Effect

In the symphony of health, the synergy effect arises as the harmonious collaboration of lifestyle components, food choices, and physiological complexities. It is not just a plain sum of parts; it is the fluid interaction where each component enhances the others, generating a collective resonance that magnifies well-being.

Picture nutrition as the melodic motif, with each nutrient having a different function in the harmonious composition. Vitamins, like musical notes, contribute to the orchestration of physiological equilibrium, each playing an essential part in cellular life. Minerals become the rhythm section, setting the pace for metabolic harmony, while macronutrients constitute the foundation, sustaining the body's energy symphony

Exercise steps onto the stage, becoming the dynamic counterpart in this health ballet. It's not only about physical exertion; it's the rhythmic cadence that resonates through the cardiovascular corridors, increasing circulation, and supporting the lively interaction of bodily systems. The synergy effect comes alive as exercise and diet join forces, forming a dynamic combination that propels the body toward optimal well-being.

Enter the mindfulness refrain—a meditation on the mental landscape that transcends stress and cultivates resilience. It's the relaxing tunes that resonate across neuronal pathways, regulating hormone balance and, in turn, impacting general wellness. The synergy effect, in this perspective, becomes the calm collaboration between mental well-being and physical vitality.

As the curtain rises on sleep, it becomes a tranquil interlude, allowing the body to heal, replenish, and prepare for the next act. The synergy effect, in this nocturnal domain, is the coordinated balance between sleep quality and general health—a silent yet powerful addition to the symphony of well-being.

Healthcare, the conductor of this symphony, becomes the guiding force, ensuring that each ingredient plays its part in harmony. Regular check-ups, preventive screenings, and appropriate interventions become the metronome, ensuring that the health symphony keeps its rhythm.

In the extensive composition of the synergy effect, there's no need for intricacy. It's a simple yet deep realization that the aspects of health—nutrition, exercise, mindfulness, and sleep—create a harmonic collaboration that transcends individual efforts. It's a symphony where each note, played in concert, contributes to the overall melody of lively well-being.

Understanding How Vitamin D, Vitamin C, and Iodine Work Together

In the symphony of nutrition, Vitamin D, Vitamin C, and Iodine appear not just as distinct performers but as a trio orchestrating an energetic collaboration that harmonizes the body's physiological rhythm. Visualize Vitamin D as the brilliant conductor, Vitamin C as the virtuoso sustaining the immunological melody, and Iodine as the silent troubadour maintaining thyroid harmony—an ensemble that transcends individual notes to produce a holistic resonance.

Vitamin D, frequently dubbed the sunshine vitamin, takes the lead in this nutritional sonata. It orchestrates calcium absorption, adds to skeletal strength, and extends its influence beyond bone health. The radiant conductor sets the setting for immunological modulation, impacting the body's defense processes and preparing the path for robust immune performance.

Enter Vitamin C, the immunological virtuoso that increases the symphony of defenses. It becomes the guardian against oxidative stress, eliminating free radicals and aiding the immune cells in their constant watch. The synergy between vitamin C and vitamin D becomes obvious as they interact in immunological orchestration, bolstering the body against foreign intruders and internal imbalances.

In this nutritional trifecta, iodine becomes the thyroid troubadour, helping to maintain metabolic equilibrium. It collaborates with the thyroid hormones, ensuring their proper synthesis and controlling the body's energy equilibrium. The modest yet crucial role of Iodine becomes clear as it weaves its impact into the metabolic symphony led by Vitamins D and C.

As the trio takes center stage, their collaborative power extends beyond individual performances. Vitamin D promotes calcium absorption, giving a basic underpinning for vitamin C's antioxidant capability and iodine's role in thyroid function. The harmony between these nutrients isn't just about individual advantages but a collective resonance that supports immune resilience, metabolic vigor, and overall well-being.

Understanding this nutritious triumvirate is not a trip into complexity but an understanding of their linked roles. It's a simple yet deep realization that in the nutritional symphony, each note—Vitamin D, Vitamin C, and Iodine—contributes to a beautiful composition that goes beyond individual performances, generating a holistic resonance in the body's orchestration of health.

Complementary Benefits for Overall Health

In the grand performance of total health, the concept of complementary benefits emerges as a symphony where multiple aspects harmonize, generating a holistic resonance that transcends individual notes. Picture this health orchestra where nutrition, exercise, and mental well-being become instrumental performers, each contributing to a lyrical composition that resonates through the body's physiological landscape.

Enter nutrition as the conductor—a maestro that orchestrates a symphony of vitamins, minerals, and macronutrients. Vitamin D takes the lead, affecting immunological strength and bone vitality, while Vitamin C becomes the virtuoso, weaving its antioxidant magic. Iodine gently ensures thyroid balance. Their collaborative influence extends beyond individual performances, generating a nutritious song that fortifies the body's defenses, sustains metabolic homeostasis, and adds to overall well-being.

Exercise steps onto the stage as the rhythmic companion. It's not just about physical activity; it's the cadence that resonates through the cardiovascular corridors, promoting circulation and enhancing metabolic vitality. The complementing tango between nutrition and exercise becomes obvious as they coordinate, forming a powerful pair that propels the body toward optimal health.

In the mental well-being overture, mindfulness becomes the calming refrain—a meditation on the mental landscape that transcends stress and cultivates resilience. The complimentary dance of mental well-being with nutrition and exercise creates a calm partnership that regulates hormone balance and affects overall health. It's a silent yet deep addition to the symphony of well-being.

Sleep becomes the peaceful pause in this health formula, allowing the body to repair, rejuvenate, and prepare for the next act. It's the silent but vital note that contributes to the overall balance of health. The complementing effects of regular sleep with nutrition, exercise, and mental well-being produce a nocturnal cadence that supports the body's physiological rhythm.

As the healthcare conductor takes the lead, regular check-ups, preventive screenings, and timely interventions become the metronome, ensuring that each element plays its role in harmony. It's a collaborative effort where nutrition, exercise, mental well-being, and healthcare coincide, generating a symphony of complementing advantages that resound through the grand performance of total health.

Creating a Balanced Nutritional Strategy

In the pursuit of a balanced nutritional plan, consider your plate as a canvas where varied hues represent a spectrum of nutrients. The key is not simply variety but intentional composition—a symphony of proteins, carbs, healthy fats, vitamins, and minerals. This nutritional orchestra plays a key role in maintaining bodily functions, improving general health, and providing the energy required for daily activities.

Begin with the foundation—an array of nutritious foods that form the cornerstone of your nutritional plan. Embrace leafy greens, colorful veggies, entire grains, lean proteins, and sources of healthy fats. These components, like instrumental players, offer unique notes to the nutritional melody, assuring a broad range of important nutrients.

Consider portion management as the tempo regulator in this dietary composition. It's not just about what's on the plate, but how much of it is consumed. Portion awareness avoids overindulgence, preserving the delicate balance essential for good health. Picture it as a conductor guiding the symphony, ensuring that each instrument plays its part without overshadowing the others.

Diversify your nutrient intake by adopting a variety of dietary categories. This nutritional harmony ensures that you obtain the benefits of different vitamins, minerals, and antioxidants. It's analogous to having a well-rounded ensemble where each section contributes to the overall richness of the song.

Integrate the principle of balance into meals. Include a combination of macronutrients—proteins, carbs, and fats—in each meal. This trio creates the backbone of prolonged energy, promoting physical activity and metabolic well-being. It's a nutritional dance where proteins provide muscle support, carbs offer energy, and healthy fats contribute to overall satiety.

Hydration becomes the hydrating refrain, an often ignored but crucial element of a balanced nutritional plan. Water, like a silent note, regulates digestion, nutrient absorption, and overall physiological processes. The orchestration of a well-hydrated body is crucial for sustaining health and supporting numerous physiological functions.

In this nutritional symphony, moderation plays a vital part. It's not about tight diets or restrictions, but about creating a rhythm that corresponds with your specific requirements and aspirations. A balanced dietary plan is durable, adaptive, and follows the body's cues, producing a happy and healthy relationship with food.

Chapter 5

Signs of Deficiency and How to Address Them

When it comes to maintaining optimal health, it is crucial to be able to recognize the indicators of a nutritional shortage. Vitamin D deficiency may appear as weariness, bone discomfort, muscle weakness, and reduced immunological function. An evaluation of your vitamin D levels can be determined through a blood test if you experience these symptoms. In order to treat the deficiency, it is necessary to expose the affected individual to sunlight, make adjustments to their diet, and, if required, take supplements under the supervision of a qualified medical practitioner.

Scurvy, often known as a deficit in vitamin C, is characterized by symptoms such as weariness, weakness in the muscles, discomfort in the joints, and swollen gums. Incorporating vitamin C-rich foods like citrus fruits, strawberries, and bell peppers into your diet is vital. Supplements may be important for people at risk, such as individuals with limited access to fresh vegetables or specific medical conditions.

Both goiter and hypothyroidism are examples of thyroid-related conditions that can be brought on by a lack of iodine. Fatigue, weight gain, and sensitivity to cold are some of the symptoms that may be experienced. Including in your diet items that are high in iodine, such as seaweed, salmon, and dairy products, can assist in the treatment of minor deficits. Individuals who are experiencing severe symptoms may be advised by a medical expert to take iodine supplements.

Many people, particularly women, suffer from iron deficiency, which manifests itself in symptoms such as weariness, weakness, and a pale complexion. Including foods that are high in iron, such as lean meats, beans, and dark leafy greens, in your diet is quite important. Iron supplements may be essential; however, consultation with a healthcare expert is advised to determine the proper amount.

Omega-3 fatty acid insufficiency may cause dry skin, brittle hair, and joint pain. Including fatty fish, flaxseeds, and walnuts in your diet can help correct this shortage. Omega-3 supplements may be indicated for people with limited dietary sources, but moderation is crucial to avoid excessive ingestion.

Recognizing these indications and treating deficits promptly is vital for general well-being. However, self-diagnosis and excessive dosage might lead to harmful effects. Seeking help from healthcare specialists ensures a targeted approach to fixing weaknesses while avoiding potential consequences.

Recognizing Symptoms of Vitamin D, Vitamin C, and Iodine Deficiency

Vitamin D, frequently referred to as the sunshine vitamin, plays a key role in different body activities. Recognizing indications of insufficiency is critical for timely intervention. Common indications include prolonged weariness, muscle weakness, and bone pain. Individuals may experience greater susceptibility to infections, and in severe cases, bone abnormalities may ensue. Deficiency can develop discreetly, making it crucial to be aware of these symptoms, especially in people with minimal solar exposure or specific health issues.

Vitamin C deficiency, known as scurvy, can result in different symptoms impacting both physical and dental health. Fatigue, muscle weakness, and joint discomfort are common indications. Swollen, bleeding gums, and a predisposition to bruise easily are classic oral signs. Individuals with inadequate consumption of vitamin C-rich foods, such as fruits and vegetables, may exhibit these symptoms. Early detection allows for dietary modifications and, if necessary, supplementation to treat the shortfall.

Iodine deficiency influences thyroid function, leading to symptoms such as weariness, weight gain, and sensitivity to cold. The most noticeable sign may be the development of a goiter—an enlargement of the thyroid gland. Recognizing these symptoms is critical, particularly in places where soil lacks sufficient iodine, altering the iodine level in dietary sources. Dietary adjustments, including the integration of iodine-rich foods or supplementation under medical advice, can help resolve these inadequacies.

Understanding the signs of these vitamin deficiencies encourages individuals to make proactive efforts toward optimal health. While some symptoms may be modest, chronic fatigue, changes in dental health, and thyroid-related disorders may warrant additional study. Consultation with healthcare professionals is vital for accurate diagnosis and specific intervention techniques, ensuring that inadequacies are treated successfully and in a timely way.

Strategies for Reversing Deficiencies

Addressing nutritional deficits demands a specialized and methodical strategy. For vitamin D deficiency, increased sunshine exposure is crucial. Spending time outdoors, particularly during peak sunlight hours, allows the skin to manufacture vitamin D. In circumstances where sunlight exposure is limited, dietary modifications become vital. Incorporating vitamin D-rich foods such as fatty fish, fortified dairy products, and egg yolks can contribute to raising vitamin D levels. Supplements may be suggested under the advice of a healthcare expert to ensure optimal dosage and effectiveness.

Vitamin C insufficiency can often be remedied by dietary adjustments. Including a range of fruits and vegetables, such as citrus fruits, strawberries, bell peppers, and broccoli, gives an abundance of vitamin C. For people with limited access to fresh produce, supplementation may be considered, although consultation with a healthcare expert is advised to determine the proper dosage.

Iodine insufficiency can be remedied by integrating iodine-rich foods into the diet. Seaweed, seafood, dairy products, and iodized salt are important sources. In locations where dietary iodine is persistently inadequate, iodine supplements may be advised, but again, consultation with a healthcare practitioner is needed to avoid excessive intake.

Iron insufficiency often requires multi-faceted therapy. Including iron-rich foods like lean meats, beans, and dark leafy greens is vital. Enhancing iron absorption by mixing iron-rich foods with vitamin C sources can be useful. Supplements may be important, particularly for persons with chronic deficits, although medical assistance is essential to avoid consequences.

For the omega-3 fatty acid shortage, introducing fatty fish, flaxseeds, chia seeds, and walnuts into the diet is useful. Fish oil supplements can be explored for people with limited dietary sources, but moderation is crucial to prevent excessive ingestion.

In all circumstances, monitoring symptoms and nutrient levels through regular check-ups is vital. Healthcare experts play a vital role in guiding clients toward successful ways of correcting deficits, guaranteeing a balanced and tailored approach to nutritional well-being.

Preventative Measures for Long-Term Health

Proactively safeguarding long-term health includes adopting a diverse approach that encompasses lifestyle choices, food habits, and preventive healthcare treatments. Regular physical activity has a key role in preventing a plethora of health conditions. Engaging in both cardiovascular and strength-building exercises not only promotes physical fitness but also contributes to metabolic health, bone density, and mental well-being. The constant integration of exercise into one's routine creates a cornerstone for long-term health.

A balanced and nutrient-rich diet is crucial in preventing nutritional deficiencies and fostering general well-being. Emphasizing entire foods, including a variety of fruits, vegetables, lean proteins, and whole grains, ensures a diverse intake of critical nutrients. Limiting the consumption of processed foods, refined carbohydrates, and excessive saturated fats is similarly crucial. This nutritional balance supports weight control, cardiovascular health, and immunological function, establishing a basis for prolonged health.

Regular health check-ups serve as a proactive technique for the early detection and prevention of any health disorders. Routine testing for problems such as blood pressure, cholesterol levels, and blood glucose provides vital insights into cardiovascular health and metabolic status. Age-appropriate screens for cancer, bone density, and other health indicators enable timely interventions, helping to prevent chronic diseases.

Mental well-being is a vital part of long-term health. Incorporating stress management practices, such as mindfulness, meditation, or indulging in hobbies, increases mental resilience. Adequate sleep, an often ignored yet crucial component, allows the body to replenish and adds to cognitive performance, emotional well-being, and general vigor.

Avoiding tobacco usage and regulating alcohol use are key lifestyle decisions for long-term health. These preventative practices dramatically reduce the risk of several chronic disorders, including cardiovascular diseases and some malignancies. Consistent hydration, maintaining a healthy body weight, and avoiding excessive sun exposure further contribute to a holistic plan for long-term well-being.

In essence, preventative strategies for long-term health comprise a proactive and aware approach to lifestyle, nutrition, and healthcare. By creating behaviors that support physical, mental, and emotional health, individuals can lay the framework for a robust and vibrant existence across the years. Regular self-care, informed lifestyle choices, and engagement with healthcare professionals build the foundation for a healthy and rewarding journey.

Chapter 6

Optimizing Your Health Routine

Optimizing your health routine entails a thoughtful and intentional approach to lifestyle decisions that contribute to overall well-being. Begin by building a balanced and nutritious diet that matches your particular needs. Prioritize a range of nutritious foods, including fruits, vegetables, lean meats, and whole grains. This nutritional basis ensures a broad intake of critical nutrients, boosting energy and supporting numerous physical functions.

Incorporating regular physical activity is crucial for optimizing health. Engage in a combination of aerobic exercises, strength training, and flexibility activities. This holistic approach not only boosts cardiovascular health and muscular strength but also contributes to bone density and general physical resilience. Tailor your exercise regimen to your interests and health goals, ensuring consistency over time.

Prioritize mental well-being as an intrinsic component of your health regimen. Incorporate stress management practices such as mindfulness, meditation, or relaxation exercises. Cultivate hobbies and activities that provide delight and relaxation. Adequate sleep is equally vital, as it directly improves cognitive function, emotional resilience, and general mental health. A consistent sleep habit supports your body's natural rhythms and contributes to healthy well-being.

Regular health check-ups and tests represent a proactive element of your health improvement approach. Schedule routine visits with healthcare providers to monitor vital health metrics such as blood pressure, cholesterol levels, and blood glucose. Age-appropriate tests for malignancies, bone health, and other disorders enable early identification and intervention, contributing to long-term health optimization.

Hydration is a fundamental yet often overlooked part of health optimization. Ensure appropriate water intake throughout the day to support numerous physiological functions, including digestion, food absorption, and temperature regulation. Consistent hydration is foundational for overall health and vigor.

Consider adopting positive lifestyle behaviors such as avoiding tobacco usage and minimizing alcohol consumption. These choices greatly contribute to long-term health optimization by minimizing the risk of chronic diseases. Limiting exposure to environmental pollutants and practicing sun protection further contribute to a balanced health regimen.

In building your health routine, it's crucial to adapt it according to your specific needs, tastes, and goals. By embracing a holistic approach incorporating nutrition, physical exercise, mental well-being, and preventative healthcare measures, you establish a blueprint for enhancing your health and cultivating a robust and vibrant existence.

Incorporating Sun Exposure Safely for Vitamin D

Incorporating sun exposure properly is a fundamental component of ensuring adequate vitamin D levels, an Essent nutrient for different physiological activities. Striking a balance between getting the benefits of sunshine and avoiding potential harm demands conscious activities. Aim for moderate sun exposure, often around 10 to 30 minutes a few times a week, depending on factors like skin type, location, and time of day. This length permits the skin to produce vitamin D without overexposing it to damaging ultraviolet (UV) rays.

Choose favorable times for sun exposure, often during the early morning or late afternoon when UVB rays are less powerful. This decreases the danger of skin injury while still facilitating vitamin D synthesis. Avoid extended sun exposure during peak hours when the sun's rays are highest, often between 10 a.m. and 4 p.m.

Consider skin type and sensitivity before exposing your skin to sunlight. Fair-skinned people may require less time in the sun compared to those with darker complexions. Use sunscreen on sections of the skin not exposed to the sun or when prolonged exposure is inevitable. Select a broad-spectrum sunscreen with an appropriate Sun Protection Factor (SPF) to protect against both UVA and UVB radiation.

Embrace a holistic approach to sun exposure by wearing protective apparel, such as hats and long sleeves, especially during lengthy time outdoors. This minimizes direct exposure and lessens the risk of sunburn. Keep in mind that elements like altitude, cloud cover, and pollution can alter UV ray intensity, requiring adjustments in sun exposure protocols accordingly.

For people with limited sun exposure or those dwelling in regions with less sunlight, dietary sources of vitamin D become crucial. Consist of fatty fish, fortified dairy products, and egg yolks in your diet. Supplements may be considered under the advice of a healthcare practitioner to achieve vitamin D requirements, particularly for people with specific health issues or those at risk of deficiency.

By incorporating sun exposure safely, individuals can harness the benefits of vitamin D production while reducing the possible hazards associated with excessive sun exposure. This balanced approach improves general health and ensures that the body obtains adequate vitamin D for numerous physiological activities.

Creating a Vitamin C-Rich Diet Plan

Creating a Vitamin C-rich meal plan is a proactive step towards maintaining general health and preventing deficits. Vitamin C, commonly known as ascorbic acid, is necessary for several body activities, including collagen formation, immune system support, and antioxidant protection.

Start by integrating a variety of fruits and vegetables into your everyday meals. Citrus fruits such as oranges, lemons, and grapefruits are well-known sources of Vitamin C. Berries, like strawberries, blueberries, and raspberries, are also wonderful alternatives. These fruits not only give Vitamin C but also contribute extra antioxidants and fiber, increasing the total nutritional profile.

Include a range of veggies in your diet, focusing on those rich in Vitamin C. Bell peppers, both red and green, are particularly high in Vitamin C concentration. Broccoli, Brussels sprouts, and cauliflower are cruciferous vegetables that deliver a considerable amount of this crucial vitamin. Leafy greens such as spinach and kale also contribute to your daily Vitamin C consumption.

Consider adding tropical fruits like pineapple and mango to your diet. These fruits not only infuse a pleasant taste but also supply a large amount of Vitamin C. Additionally, they give a natural sweetness that might fulfill cravings for sugary treats.

Opt for fresh or less processed types of fruits and vegetables whenever feasible, as cooking can occasionally diminish Vitamin C concentration. However, steaming or microwaving veggies can help retain more of this water-soluble vitamin compared to boiling.

Incorporate Vitamin C-rich foods into multiple meals and snacks throughout the day to ensure constant consumption. For example, add slices of strawberries to your morning yogurt, including a colorful salad with lunch, and enjoy a fruit smoothie as an afternoon snack.

If dietary restrictions or preferences limit your ability to consume Vitamin C-rich foods, consider supplementation under the advice of a healthcare expert. Supplements can be an efficient approach to ensuring you achieve your daily requirements, especially if dietary sources are insufficient.

By constructing a Vitamin C-rich meal plan that includes a varied assortment of fruits and vegetables, you not only increase your general health but also create a delightful and enjoyable method to reach your nutritional needs.

Iodine Supplementation and Dietary Guidelines

Iodine is an essential ingredient for thyroid health, and ensuring enough consumption is vital to prevent shortages and related health complications. While many persons may acquire sufficient iodine through food sources, supplementation may be necessary in some conditions. It is crucial to stick to established dietary standards and recognize when supplementation is suitable.

Dietary items rich in iodine include seaweed, salmon, dairy products, and iodized salt. Including these foods in your normal diet aids in maintaining appropriate iodine levels. However, factors such as regional variations in soil iodine content and dietary preferences may alter the availability of iodine-rich foods.

Pregnant women, in particular, have increased iodine requirements due to the essential function iodine plays in fetal brain development. Therefore, healthcare experts typically recommend iodine supplementation throughout pregnancy to ensure both maternal and fetal iodine needs are satisfied. Consultation with a healthcare practitioner is important to identify the optimum dosage and duration of supplementation.

Individuals living in places with low soil iodine content may suffer an increased risk of iodine shortage. In such circumstances, healthcare experts may offer iodine supplementation to offset this geographical difference. However, it is necessary to check with a healthcare expert before commencing supplementation, since excessive iodine intake can have harmful effects on thyroid function.

Maintaining a balanced approach to iodine consumption entails being cognizant of both dietary sources and prospective supplements. Striking this equilibrium ensures that iodine levels coincide with suggested standards without causing deficits or excessive ingestion. Regular health check-ups and talks with healthcare experts play a crucial role in adapting iodine recommendations to individual needs and circumstances.

adhering to dietary standards that contain iodine-rich foods is a crucial strategy for maintaining adequate iodine levels. In specific instances, such as pregnancy or dwelling in locations with limited iodine availability, supplementation may be necessary, however, this decision should be taken in cooperation with a healthcare practitioner to ensure safe and efficient iodine management.

Chapter 7

Lifestyle Factors and Healthful Habits

Lifestyle factors and healthful practices have an important impact in defining general well-being and preventing numerous health concerns. Regular physical activity is a cornerstone of a healthful lifestyle. Engaging in a combination of aerobic exercises, strength training, and flexibility activities adds to cardiovascular health, muscle strength, and overall physical resilience. It is crucial to discover activities that correspond with personal interests and integrate them consistently into everyday routines.

Dietary choices greatly impact health outcomes. Adopting a balanced and healthy diet that includes a range of fruits, vegetables, lean proteins, and whole grains delivers important nutrients that support biological functioning. Limiting the consumption of processed foods, sweets, and excessive saturated fats is vital for maintaining a nutritious diet. Hydration also serves a key role, supporting many physiological processes and boosting general health.

Adequate sleep is a core beneficial habit that sometimes gets forgotten. Establishing consistent sleep practices and receiving sufficient rest each night is critical for cognitive function, emotional well-being, and physical recovery. Quality sleep adds to overall vigor and resilience.

Stress management is another crucial part of a healthy lifestyle. Chronic stress can significantly influence both physical and mental health. Using stress-reducing activities such as mindfulness, meditation, or indulging in hobbies builds emotional resilience and supports mental well-being.

Avoiding tobacco usage and regulating alcohol consumption are crucial healthful practices. These lifestyle choices dramatically reduce the risk of several chronic disorders, including cardiovascular diseases and certain malignancies. Additionally, they contribute to increased respiratory and general organ health.

Sun safety is vital to prevent skin damage and lower the risk of skin cancer. Using sunscreen, wearing protective clothes, and avoiding prolonged sun exposure during peak hours contribute to a healthful approach to enjoying outdoor activities.

Regular health check-ups and preventive screenings are proactive actions that individuals can take to monitor and preserve their health. These meetings with healthcare professionals enable early detection and action, limiting the progression of potential health disorders.

Adopting healthier behaviors entails a holistic approach to lifestyle choices. By embracing regular physical activity, maintaining a balanced diet, prioritizing sleep, controlling stress, and avoiding hazardous substances, individuals can build a healthier lifestyle that promotes long-term well-being.

The Role of Exercise in Vitamin Utilization

Exercise offers a crucial function in the usage of vitamins within the human body, contributing to overall health and well-being. Physical exercise promotes the absorption and metabolism of vitamins, ensuring their efficient utilization for numerous physiological functions. One famous example is Vitamin D, which is generated in the skin in reaction to sunshine exposure during outdoor activities. Regular exercise encourages enough sun exposure, boosting the natural generation of Vitamin D and contributing to bone health and immunological function.

Engaging in aerobic workouts, such as jogging, swimming, or cycling, increases cardiovascular health and oxygenates the body. This enhanced circulation facilitates the transfer of vital vitamins, such as Vitamin C, to numerous tissues and organs. Vitamin C, recognized for its antioxidant characteristics, is necessary for collagen formation and immune system function, and its effective usage is promoted by regular aerobic exercise.

Strength training techniques, including weightlifting and resistance training, increase muscle growth and repair. This process involves the consumption of vitamins such as B-complex vitamins (B1, B2, B6, and B12) that play a critical role in energy metabolism and muscular function. Ensuring an appropriate intake of these vitamins through a balanced diet is vital for persons engaging in strength-building workouts.

Exercise-induced oxidative stress, a normal result of physical activity, shows the necessity of antioxidant vitamins. Vitamin E, found in nuts, seeds, and vegetable oils, and Vitamin A, prevalent in colored fruits and vegetables, work as antioxidants that help minimize the impact of oxidative stress on cells. Regular exercise, by boosting the body's demand for oxygen during physical effort, highlights the need for a well-balanced diet rich in these antioxidant vitamins.

Exercise promotes the usage of vitamins by enhancing their absorption, metabolism, and effective distribution to various tissues. Whether through outdoor activities supporting Vitamin D synthesis, cardiovascular exercises facilitating vitamin circulation, strength training enhancing muscle function, or antioxidant-rich diets complementing oxidative stress management, the interplay between exercise and vitamins is integral to maintaining optimal health. A well-rounded approach that involves both regular physical exercise and a balanced diet allows the harmonious usage of vitamins for overall well-being.

Stress Management and Its Impact on Nutrient Absorption

Stress management plays a crucial role in ensuring proper nutrition absorption and overall digestive health. The body's response to stress, typically described as the "fight or flight" response, can affect several physiological processes, including digestion and nutrient absorption. Chronic stress can lead to abnormalities in gastrointestinal function, decreasing the efficiency with which vital nutrients are absorbed and utilized by the body.

One substantial consequence of stress on nutritional absorption is the suppression of stomach secretion. Stress can lead to decreased stomach acid production, impacting the breakdown of food in the stomach. This may limit the absorption of important nutrients, including proteins, minerals, and vitamins. Consequently, those suffering prolonged stress may be at an increased risk of vitamin shortages.

The stress hormone cortisol, secreted during moments of heightened stress, can also alter nutrient absorption. Cortisol may interfere with the absorption of minerals such as calcium, magnesium, and zinc. Prolonged rise of cortisol levels may result in mineral imbalances that can have cascade repercussions on bone health, immunological function, and overall well-being.

In addition to influencing the physical elements of digestion, stress can influence food choices and eating behaviors. Individuals under chronic stress may be more prone to choosing less nutritious food choices or participating in emotional eating, thus lowering their overall nutritional intake.

Furthermore, stress management practices might significantly influence the body's ability to absorb and utilize nutrients. Practices such as mindfulness, deep breathing exercises, and meditation have been demonstrated to reduce stress levels and increase digestive health. By implementing stress-reduction measures into everyday routines, individuals can boost their general well-being and support proper nutritional absorption.

The connection between stress management and nutrient absorption highlights the necessity of a comprehensive approach to health. By managing stress in various ways and creating a supportive environment for digestion, individuals can maximize the absorption of critical nutrients, supporting overall health and vitality.

Quality Sleep for Overall Well-Being

Quality sleep is a vital foundation of total well-being, having a pivotal role in physical, mental, and emotional health. During sleep, the body undertakes crucial activities that contribute to cellular repair, immunological function, and cognitive consolidation. Adequate and restorative sleep is vital for sustaining overall health and resiliency.

One key part of sleep's impact on general well-being resides in its involvement in physical recuperation. Sleep is a phase during which the body heals and regenerates tissues, muscles, and numerous physiological systems. This reparative process is necessary for recovery from daily wear and tear, maintaining overall physical resilience and vitality.

Cognitive performance and memory consolidation are tightly tied to the quality of sleep. During different sleep stages, the brain analyzes and organizes information received throughout the day. This consolidation of memories and the facilitation of learning contribute to cognitive function, problem-solving ability, and overall mental sharpness.

Sleep also plays a critical function in keeping a robust immune system. Adequate and peaceful sleep stimulates the development of immune cells and antibodies, boosting the body's defenses against infections and illnesses. Chronic sleep loss, on the other hand, might weaken immune function, raising susceptibility to numerous health concerns.

Emotional well-being is tightly interwoven with sleep quality. A good night's sleep adds to mood control and emotional resiliency. Sleep deprivation, contrary, can worsen stress, anxiety, and irritability, compromising general emotional stability.

Establishing stable sleep patterns and ensuring appropriate sleep length are key to receiving the advantages of excellent sleep. Creating a sleep-conducive atmosphere, reducing exposure to electronic gadgets before bedtime, and keeping to a regular sleep schedule are practical techniques to promote restful sleep.

The value of quality sleep cannot be emphasized in the context of general well-being. Recognizing sleep as a critical component of a healthy lifestyle underlines the need to prioritize appropriate rest for optimal physical, mental, and emotional health. By understanding and practicing appropriate sleep habits, individuals can boost their general well-being and resilience in the face of life's obstacles.

Chapter 8

Special Considerations

Special considerations are necessary when addressing unique health demands and conditions. One such aspect is age, as nutritional requirements vary over the life cycle. Infants, children, adolescents, adults, and older adults have varied nutritional demands, determined by growth, development, and aging processes. Tailoring food choices to meet age-specific requirements guarantees optimal health and well-being.

Health issues and medical concerns also deserve special care. Individuals with chronic illnesses such as diabetes, cardiovascular diseases, or autoimmune disorders may require specific dietary adjustments to manage their conditions efficiently. Consultation with healthcare specialists and licensed dietitians is vital to designing tailored nutritional regimens that fit with medical demands.

Pregnancy is a unique period that involves special care for both the mother and the developing fetus. Adequate intake of vital nutrients, such as folic acid, iron, and calcium, is crucial for fetal development and maternal health. Pregnant individuals should obtain information on correct nutrition to support a healthy pregnancy and achieve optimal outcomes for both mother and child.

Cultural and culinary preferences influence food choices and nutritional practices. Recognizing and appreciating cultural diversity is crucial in offering dietary recommendations that are both healthful and culturally appropriate. Integrating traditional foods and culinary traditions into dietary programs can promote adherence and contribute to overall well-being.

Special nutritional needs may also occur in those adopting vegetarian or vegan lifestyles. Proper planning is needed to ensure that these persons acquire appropriate nutrients, such as protein, iron, calcium, and vitamin B12, which are typically present in animal products. Well-informed dietary choices and, if necessary, supplements can assist in meeting nutritional requirements in plant-based diets.

Allergies and intolerances require careful attention when developing dietary programs. Individuals with sensitivies to certain foods or chemicals must avoid these allergens to avert harmful responses. Additionally, those with intolerances, such as lactose intolerance, may need other food sources to achieve their nutritional demands without causing digestive pain.

Special considerations in nutrition involve several characteristics, including age, health issues, pregnancy, cultural preferences, dietary choices, and allergies. Tailoring nutritional counsel to fit these particular needs ensures that dietary recommendations align with personal circumstances, encouraging optimal health outcomes and overall well-being.

Vitamins and Minerals for Different Life Stages

The nutritional demands for vitamins and minerals fluctuate across distinct life phases, reflecting the dynamic requirements of growth, development, and aging. In the early stages of life, babies and children require vital nutrients to sustain rapid growth and development. Adequate intake of vitamins such as A, C, D, and minerals like iron and calcium is necessary during this age to promote good bone building, immune system development, and cognitive function.

As individuals advance into adolescence, the demand for particular nutrients intensifies due to the beginning of puberty and increased physical activity. Nutrients such as B-complex vitamins, iron, and zinc play a critical role in regulating hormonal balance, improving energy metabolism, and sustaining general well-being during this active time of life.

Pregnancy is a unique life period that poses distinct nutritional demands on both the mother and the developing fetus. Folic acid, iron, calcium, and vitamin D are particularly necessary during pregnancy to support fetal growth, avoid neural tube defects, maintain bone health, and ensure a robust immune system. Meeting these nutritional demands is crucial for the health of both the mother and the infant.

Adulthood provides its own set of nutritional requirements, affected by factors such as lifestyle, work, and overall health. Vitamins and minerals continue to be vital for sustaining optimal health and preventing chronic illnesses. For example, vitamin K and calcium become increasingly necessary for supporting bone health, while antioxidants like vitamin E and selenium support overall cellular health and protection against oxidative stress.

As individuals enter the later phases of life, especially in the older population, emphasis changes toward maintaining bone density, limiting cognitive decline, and sustaining immunological function. Adequate intake of vitamin B12, vitamin D, calcium, and omega-3 fatty acids become necessary to address common concerns such as bone health, cognitive function, and cardiovascular health in aging persons.

Recognizing the variable nutritional needs across different life phases is vital for ensuring optimal health and minimizing vitamin deficits. Tailoring dietary choices to match the specific demands of each life stage ensures that individuals acquire the necessary vitamins and minerals to promote growth, development, and overall well-being throughout their life journey.

Health Conditions and Their Impact on Nutrient Needs

Various health issues can greatly alter an individual's nutrient demands, underlining the significance of tailored dietary choices to manage and address specific health concerns. Chronic illnesses, such as diabetes, cardiovascular diseases, and autoimmune disorders, typically demand specific nutritional regimens to support optimal health and manage symptoms.

Diabetes, for example, demands close attention to carbohydrate intake to maintain blood sugar levels. Monitoring and managing the consumption of vitamins and minerals like chromium, magnesium, and B-complex vitamins are critical to improving insulin sensitivity and general metabolic function in patients with diabetes.

Cardiovascular illnesses, like hypertension and excessive cholesterol, underline the necessity of a heart-healthy diet rich in nutrients that support cardiovascular health. Nutrients including omega-3 fatty acids, potassium, and antioxidants have a crucial role in controlling blood pressure, and cholesterol levels, and lowering inflammation, contributing to overall cardiovascular well-being.

Individuals with autoimmune illnesses, such as rheumatoid arthritis or celiac disease, often benefit from dietary modifications to manage inflammation and support immunological function. Nutrients including vitamin D, omega-3 fatty acids, and antioxidants may be particularly useful in tackling the unique problems faced by autoimmune disorders.

Gastrointestinal illnesses, such as irritable bowel syndrome (IBS) or inflammatory bowel disease (IBD), can impair food absorption and digestion. Tailoring the diet to fit specific sensitivities, maintaining enough intake of important nutrients, and potentially including dietary supplements become crucial in controlling the nutritional elements of these disorders.

Nutrient demands are also greatly altered by certain life phases, and health problems can magnify these needs. Pregnancy, breastfeeding, and postmenopausal periods all bring distinct nutritional challenges and considerations. Addressing these problems demands a comprehensive approach that considers both the individual's health status and the unique life stage.

Evaluating the influence of health conditions on nutritional demands is crucial in creating successful dietary plans that support general health and well-being. Working in partnership with healthcare providers and registered dietitians is vital to establish tailored nutrition regimens that correspond with an individual's health condition, ensuring they obtain the necessary nutrients to control symptoms and promote optimal health.

Consultation with Healthcare Professionals

Consultation with healthcare professionals, particularly registered dietitians and nutritionists, is a crucial step in building a specific and effective nutritional plan. These professionals contribute a wealth of knowledge and expertise in comprehending the subtleties of individual health issues, dietary preferences, and lifestyle considerations. Through detailed assessments, they can adapt nutritional advice to match specific requirements and goals.

One of the key advantages of talking with healthcare professionals is the chance to receive evidence-based counsel. Registered dietitians and nutritionists base their recommendations on the latest scientific research, guaranteeing that dietary programs are not only beneficial but also safe for individuals with diverse health concerns. This evidence-based strategy contributes to the development of sustainable and health-promoting dietary habits.

Healthcare experts are trained to undertake complete assessments of an individual's health status, taking into account aspects such as medical history, current health issues, medications, and lifestyle. This holistic understanding enables them to deliver tailored dietary advice that incorporates the specific demands and problems of each individual.

Individuals with chronic health concerns, such as diabetes, cardiovascular diseases, or gastrointestinal disorders, might benefit considerably from the experience of healthcare professionals. These professionals can help manage particular dietary requirements connected to the disease, provide direction on portion control, and propose nutrient-dense foods to enhance overall health.

Pregnant individuals or those wanting to get pregnant also benefit from discussions with healthcare specialists, particularly in navigating the specialized nutritional demands of this life stage. Guidance on critical nutrients such as folic acid, iron, and calcium is crucial for maintaining a healthy pregnancy and good fetal growth.

Moreover, healthcare practitioners play a critical role in treating dietary concerns connected to allergies, intolerances, or dietary restrictions, ensuring that clients receive appropriate nutrition while avoiding potential allergens or triggers. This tailored method helps individuals control their food choices without compromising their nutritional well-being.

Engaging with healthcare professionals offers individuals with the skills needed to navigate the complex landscape of nutrition. Through tailored assessments, evidence-based recommendations, and a focus on individual needs, healthcare professionals contribute to the formulation of successful and sustainable dietary plans that promote optimal health and well-being.

Conclusion

In summation, studying the composition of vitamins and minerals, their roles in different life stages, and their impact on health issues highlights the significance of individualized nutrition. The dynamic combination of individual demands, health state, and lifestyle necessitates a comprehensive approach to food choices. Throughout this journey, the value of consulting with healthcare professionals, particularly registered dietitians and nutritionists, has been underlined as important in designing individualized dietary regimens.

Understanding the varied nutritional demands at distinct life phases is vital for ensuring good health and minimizing deficits. From the early stages of infancy and childhood, through the active years of youth and adulthood, to the considerations of pregnancy and the challenges of aging, identifying the individual dietary requirements is vital for supporting well-being.

Health issues further underline the necessity for a tailored approach to diet. Chronic illnesses, immunological disorders, gastrointestinal troubles, and cardiovascular concerns all require specific dietary regimens to manage symptoms, promote overall health, and prevent consequences. The intricate link between health issues and dietary needs underlines the need for evidence-based counsel from healthcare providers.

Consultation with healthcare professionals emerges as a cornerstone in the formulation of successful and sustainable nutritional regimens. These specialists bring a thorough grasp of individual health, delivering evidence-based suggestions that correspond with specific conditions, dietary limitations, and lifestyle preferences. Their experience proves useful in addressing the varied facets of diet and supporting long-term health.

As individuals navigate the terrain of food options, addressing the role of vitamins and minerals becomes crucial in creating a balanced and nutritious nutritional plan. This conclusion serves as a reminder that the quest for optimal health via nutrition is a continuing journey, one that benefits from the advice of healthcare professionals and a commitment to informed and thoughtful dietary choices. Ultimately, the combination of individualized nutrition and professional experience sets the foundation for a healthier and more resilient existence.

Recap of Key Takeaways

Throughout our studies of vitamins and minerals, several major conclusions have emerged, shining light on the pivotal role these micronutrients play in supporting good health. Firstly, the realization that distinct life stages come with particular nutritional demands highlights the significance of adjusting dietary choices to satisfy specific needs. From infancy to the old years, knowing and adapting to these requirements contribute to general well-being.

Health issues further underline the need for an individualized diet. Chronic illnesses, immunological disorders, and gastrointestinal issues demand specific nutritional solutions. This underscores the delicate relationship between individual health state and dietary demands, underlining the usefulness of a personalized approach in controlling symptoms and promoting overall health.

The synergistic impact of vitamins and minerals, notably the dynamic trio of Vitamin D, Vitamin C, and Iodine, has been a repeating theme. These micronutrients not only fulfill independent jobs but also collaborate to boost each other's functions. Recognizing this interplay is crucial in building a comprehensive nutritional approach that harnesses the combined benefits for maximum health.

The role of sunshine in Vitamin D production has been stressed, highlighting the natural and major supply of this crucial vitamin. Understanding the significance of sunshine and its impact on overall health further highlights the holistic approach required in addressing nutritional needs.

Consultation with healthcare professionals, particularly licensed dietitians and nutritionists, stands out as a cornerstone in the pursuit of optimal health. Their experience, built-in evidence-based techniques, ensures that nutritional regimens are not only effective but also safe, addressing specific health issues, dietary restrictions, and lifestyle choices.

As we summarize these major lessons, it becomes obvious that a balanced nutritional plan entails more than just achieving fundamental dietary requirements. It incorporates a comprehensive understanding of individual needs, the dynamic aspect of health, and the synergistic effects of vitamins and minerals. In this continual journey towards optimal health, the integration of professional assistance and informed food choices forms the bedrock for sustained well-being.

Appendix

Supplemental Information on Vitamin D, Vitamin C, and Iodine

Supplemental information on Vitamin D, Vitamin C, and Iodine provides a deeper understanding of these vital micronutrients and their specialized functions in supporting general health. Vitamin D, frequently referred to as the "sunshine vitamin," plays a crucial function in bone health by assisting in the absorption of calcium. It is vital for the control of immunological function and has been connected with several health advantages, including lowering the risk of certain chronic diseases.

Vitamin C, known for its antioxidant effects, extends beyond its reputation for aiding the immune system. This water-soluble vitamin plays a critical role in collagen formation, wound healing, and the protection of cells from oxidative stress. It also promotes the absorption of non-heme iron from plant-based diets, adding to the overall iron balance in the body.

Iodine, a frequently neglected but crucial trace element, is fundamental for thyroid function. It is a fundamental component of thyroid hormones, which control metabolism and play a significant role in growth and development. Iodine shortage can lead to thyroid issues and significantly impair cognitive development, making it vital to guarantee an appropriate intake of this mineral.

Understanding the sources of these vitamins and minerals is crucial to maintaining a well-balanced diet. While sunshine is a natural source of Vitamin D, dietary sources such as fatty fish, fortified meals, and supplements contribute to meeting prescribed levels. Vitamin C is abundant in fruits and vegetables, with citrus fruits, strawberries, bell peppers, and broccoli being significant sources. Iodine is typically found in iodized salt, seafood, dairy products, and seaweed.

Supplementation may be necessary to treat deficits or meet specific health demands. Vitamin D supplementation is commonly suggested, especially for persons with limited sun exposure or those at risk of deficiency. Vitamin C supplements can be advantageous for persons with inadequate dietary consumption, particularly during periods of heightened physiological stress. Iodine supplementation may be explored in countries where dietary iodine is insufficient or for persons with specific medical issues.

It is vital to highlight that while supplements can be useful, they should be used wisely, and consultation with healthcare specialists is advisable. Excessive intake of some vitamins and minerals might have detrimental effects, stressing the significance of tailored counsel to guarantee safe and effective supplementation.

Additional Resources for Further Reading

For readers eager to go deeper into the subject of vitamins and minerals, there are various credible sites available for further study. Scientific journals such as the "American Journal of Clinical Nutrition," "Journal of the American Medical Association," and "Nutrients" provide comprehensive insights into the latest research findings, ensuring access to evidence-based information on the roles, benefits, and potential risks associated with Vitamin D, Vitamin C, and Iodine.

Renowned health organizations are great sources of credible information. The World Health Organization (WHO), the National Institutes of Health (NIH), and the Centers for Disease Control and Prevention (CDC) offer a wealth of data on recommended daily intakes, health implications of deficiencies, and guidelines for achieving optimal levels of these essential micronutrients.

Books authored by acknowledged professionals in nutrition and healthcare can provide in-depth knowledge and practical recommendations. Titles such "The Vitamin D Solution" by Michael F. Horlick, "Curing the Incurable: Vitamin C,

Infectious Diseases, and Toxins" by Thomas E. Levy, and "Iodine: Why You Need It, Why You Can't Live Without It" by David Brownstein offer valuable insights into the roles of these micronutrients and their impact on health.

Educational websites created by respectable universities can be valuable resources for accessible and reliable information. Websites such as the Mayo Clinic, WebMD, and the Linus Pauling Institute offer a plethora of information on vitamins and minerals, including their functions, dietary sources, and potential health benefits.

Podcasts and webinars with professionals in the field of nutrition give an entertaining and educational method to stay updated on the latest research and trends. Platforms such as TED Talks typically offer talks by top researchers and healthcare practitioners discussing various elements of nutrition and its impact on health.

Engaging with these resources not only broadens one's grasp of the subject area but also assures that the information received is anchored in scientific rigor and expert consensus. As the subject of nutrition continues to grow, remaining informed through different and reliable sources is vital to making well-informed judgments regarding one's health and dietary choices.